100 Physical Education Activities

DENIS O'DRISCOLL

BOCA RATON PUBLIC LIBRARY
BOCA RATON, FLORIDA

Copyright © 2021 by Denis O'Driscoll

All rights reserved. This book or any portion thereof may not be reproduced or transmitted in any form or manner, electronic or mechanical, including photocopying, recording, or by any information storage or retrieval system, without the express written permission of the copyright owner except for the use of brief quotations in a book review or other noncommercial uses permitted by copyright law.

Printed in the United States of America

Library of Congress Control Number:		2020923068
ISBN:	Softcover	978-1-64908-567-2
	eBook	978-1-64908-566-5
	Hardback	978-1-64908-733-1

Republished by: PageTurner Press and Media LLC
Publication Date: 01/04/2021

To order copies of this book, contact:
PageTurner Press and Media
Phone: 1-888-447-9651
order@pageturner.us
www.pageturner.us

100 Physical Education Activities

No child should be robbed of the joy which can be

found in skilful

Bodily movement, of the social contacts it can

provide during the

Pre-adolescent and adolescent periods,

or of the contribution

Which adequate exercise and bodily expression

can make to the

General mental as well as physical health and

Vigor throughout life.

Marian E Breckenridge and E Lee Vincent,

Child Development, WB Saunders and Co.,

Philadelphia, 1943

Preface

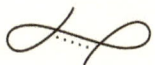

These activities are child-centered – simple, safe, enjoyable and need no equipment.

It is commendable to continue to emphasize the importance of physical education's place in the curriculum. The benefits of PE carry over to other disciplines and contribute to the formation of a well-educated individual. This book takes in twelve years of experience as an Irish national teacher.

I obtained my information from:

School Work, St. Patrick's College of Education, Dublin, 1966

Planning the Programme, Physical Education in the Primary School, Part Two, Ministry of Education, Her Majesty's Stationery Office, London, 1959

Physical Activities for the Primary Grades, Department of Education of the Province of Nova Scotia, Canada, 1960

Ghary M Akers, *Elementary Physical Education Activities,* Alabama State Department of Education, Montgomery, 1984

Physical Education in Oregon Schools, Oregon Department of Education, Salem, Oregon, 1979

Aids in Physical Education for Physical Education and Classroom Teachers, State Department of Education, Santa Fe, New Mexico, 1968

THE ACTIVITIES

1. AROUND BALL

Roll the ball in a continuous circle around the stomach and back as fast as you can.

2. BACK TO BACK

Child and partner stand back to back, interlocking their elbows. Alternatively lean forward slowly lifting the relaxed partner on his back and then return to the original position. Repeat the activity with the relaxed partner now learning forward.

3. BALLOON DANCE

Have two students place an inflated balloon between their waists or foreheads. They then dance to slow music or perform various activities without dropping the balloon.

4. BALLOONS

The children are the balloons, and at first are deflated (lying on the floor). The teacher slowly stands and become as large and wide as possible. The air may be let out slowly or with a sudden 'pop'.

5. BALLOON VOLLEYBALL

Play volleyball using a balloon for the ball and a rope or chairs for the net. Balloon may be hit any number of times.

6. BEAR WALK

Place hands on floor with arms and knees straight. Body sways from side to side as a lumbering bear would walk.

7. BELLS

Jump into air and click heels together, first to the left, then to the right. Add double click if possible.

8. BICYCLES

Lie on the back with the legs raised high in the air. Move the legs and knees to resemble riding a bicycle. This exercise should not be done too quickly.

9. BLIND BALANCE

Heels together. Stand up on toes. Close eyes. Hold position for ten seconds.

10. BLOW BALL

To increase lung capacity, ask the child to try to blow a light ball or piece of paper from one side of the room to the other, while crawling after it.

11. BOUNCE

Stand erect, feet comfortable width apart and hands on hips. Jump up and down on balls of the feet for the duration of sixteen bounces.

12. BRIDGES

Children place hands on the floor and make a 'high' bridge to let tall sailing boats pass underneath. "Now make a bridge over a wide,

wide river". "Can you think of any other way to make a bridge?"

13. BUCKETBALL

Two buckets on the ground as goals. A restraining circle may be drawn around each bucket. Same rules as basketball.

14. BULL ON THE MAT

All players on hands and knees on mat, push other off mat, last one is the bull.

15. CAMEL WALK

Bend forward, cross arms in back to make a camel's hump. Walk slowly, first swinging the head high, then low. Lie down to rest without folding arms.

16. CAT WALK

All fours position. Lean forward till chest is a few inches from the floor and creep forward.

17. CHINESE BOXING

Partners standing facing each other, each grasping the opponent's left wrist with right hand. Each trying to hit the other with the left hand.

18. CHINESE GET-UP

Partners stand back-to-back with elbows locked. Sink to floor and rise by taking small walking steps and pressing against backs. Partners should be about the same size. It may be advised to have boys work with boys and girls work with girls.

19. CLOCK PENDULUM

Stand with feet apart, hands on hips, bend trunk from side to side. Children may repeat 'tick-tock'. Movement should only be sideways, not forward and backward.

20. COFFEE GRINDER

Place one hand on the floor, stretch both legs sideways. Taking all the weight on one hand and arm, walk all the way round the hand keeping the body as straight as possible.

21. COME TO THE CIRCUS

The children imitate different animals as called by the ringmaster who stands in the centre. Some ideas for the movement interpretation are – elephant, kangaroo, tiger, pony, dog, etc.

22. CRAB BALL

Court approximately 25'x30'. Players in crab position try to kick ball over opponent's goal line for one point. Fifteen points is game.

23. CRAB WALK

From a sitting position the child raises his body off the ground so that his weight is supported by hands and feet. The stomach is raised as high as possible and the face is pointed upward. The child then walks forward and backward in this position a distance of 10 to 20 feet.

24. CRAZY MOVER

Stand and place one leg around the other. Move slightly forward and backward in this manner.

25. DOASIDO

As child says, "Do as I do", he makes a movement, such as hopping, running or an animal walk, and all must follow his movement. Choose a new leader then.

26. DODGE BALL

The children form a circle, one child in the centre. The children roll the ball back and forth trying to hit the feet of the centre child. When hit the child leaves the circle and the child that rolled the ball successfully goes in the centre.

27. DOG RUN

On all fours, running in various directions, occasionally placing legs outside and ahead of both hands which are on the floor indication a fast dog run.

28. DUAL BASKETBALL

Two balls in play at once. Forces team to use man-to-man defense. Opposing team puts the ball back into play immediately after a goal has been scored.

29. DUCK WADDLE

Squat, place hands on knees, waddle forward.

30. FOOT FENCING

Standing on one foot, using the other foot to over-balance the opponent.

31. FREE TAG

One or two players are chosen to chase the others. If a player is touched he becomes "He" and the game continues without a pause.

32. FROGS

Hands on the floor and arms between the knees. Jump forward, kicking legs to the rear. In the jumping action hands must be moved forward. To avoid bruising hands, a smooth place should be selected.

33. GREET THE TOE

Stand on one foot; grasp the other foot at the arch with two hands. Bend forward and at the same time lift the foot, attempting to touch the toe to the forehead or nose.

34. HAND WRESTLE

Clasp right hand of opponent and pull off balance.

35. HEAD BALANCE

Equipment: book or small pebble. Stand with object balanced on head. Walk, and then sit down, without dropping the object.

36. HEAD BALL

Crawling on hands and feet, the child pushes a ball with his head and rolls it along the ground.

37. HIGH KICK

Stand in place; kick as high as possible.

38. HUG KNEES

Stand on one leg, bring the other knee up to chest, and hug it close. Balance while counting 5. Repeat with other leg.

39. HUMAN ARCH

Lie on the back, and arch the body to the rest on head and feet.

40. HUMAN TOP

Jump, make a half, three-quarter or full turn, and in good balance.

41. INCH WORM

Starting from a standing position, the child bends forward and places both hands on the floor. The feet are kept stationary while the hands walk forward as far as possible. Then the hands remain stationary while the feet walk forward to a position close to the hands. The cycle is then repeated.

42. JUMP TOE TOUCH

Jump into the air, extend legs sideward and slightly forward. Touch hands to toes.

43. KANGAROO HOP

Use a small ball to hold between the knees. Hop forward without dropping the ball. May be used in relay drills.

44. KEEP THE BALL MOVING

The players arrange themselves in small groups with a ball to each group. On a given signal they move about passing the ball from one to another as speedily as they can.

45. KNEE BOXING

Working in pairs, each one trying to slap the knees of his opponent. Three rounds of fifteen seconds each. Winner is one who scores most hits during this period.

46. LAME DOG WALK

On all fours, raise one foot in the air and walk as a dog on three legs.

47. LAST MAN OVER

Players race to goal and try to keep others from arriving there first, even if they have to push, shove, etc.

48. LEG TUG OF WAR

Partners stand facing each other with right legs raised forward and feet interlocked behind ankles. They use this leg grip to pull each other.

49. MONKEY RUN

On all fours scamper agilely, imitating a monkey. Put down hands, then feet.

50. MULE KICK

Bend forward, place hands on floor, bend knees and kick into air as mule.

51. NECK PULL

Partners clasp fingers behind the opponent's neck. Each tries to pull the other four yards.

52. OBSTINATE CALF

Children work in pairs. One goes down on all fours. The second child puts both hands around the calf's neck and tries to pull forward the calf that strongly resists.

53. ONE ARM SUPPORT

Push up position, and then sideways, balancing on one arm.

54. ONE FOOT STAND

Stand on one foot, hands clasped over the head, eyes closed. Hold this position as long as possible without moving the foot.

55. ONE LEG FOOTBALL

Two balls in play at once.

56. PAPER STEPPING STONES

Each player goes down and back moving the paper stones in order to walk.

57. PIGGYBACK RELAY

Player 1 piggybacks player 2 to the turning line about 20 or 30 feet away. Player 2 runs back to the starting line and piggybacks player 3 to the turning line. The relay continues until all the players have crossed the turning line.

58. PRISONER

Circle formation with "It" inside circle of clasped hands. "It" tries to break through circle.

59. RABBIT RUN

The child puts his hands together on the ground with his knees bent and his feet close to his hands. He moves both his hands forward and then quickly brings his feet up to his hands with a small jump. Try slowly and then faster.

60. ROCKING CHAIR

Sit down on edge of mat on floor. Bring knees to chest and hold with arms. Rock on to back and then to feet, keeping the crouched position.

61. ROMAN WRESTLE

Rider on horse who is on hands and knees. Riders wrestle each other off their mounts.

62. RUN AND SWING

Swing on heavy rope which is fastened to a high strong limb of a tree.

63. SCRAMBLE BALL

Free-for-all scrambles for tossed ball.

64. SEAL CRAWL

Place hands (flippers) on floor, shoulder width apart. Legs drag behind. Move forward taking all the weight on the hands and arms. Keep child's back as straight as possible.

65. SEWING MACHINE

Running in place, hands on hips, start slowly and lightly. Increase speed gradually.

66. SHADOWS

Children work in pairs. One child tries to

stand on another child's shadow as they run a play area on a sunny day.

67. SHOULDER PUSH

Partners put hands on each other's shoulders. First person to push the other out of the circle wins.

68. SHRUGGING SHOULDERS

Shrug left shoulder up and down 10 times. Right shoulder 10 times. Both 10 times.

69. SIAMESE TWINS

Partners stand back-to-back and hook elbows. One walks forward and the other walks backwards.

70. SINGLE JET

Stand on one leg and on it balance the body in the shape of a cross, parallel to the floor.

71. SIT AND RISE

Child lies on the ground and rises off it with

the arms lifted up behind. Keep the body straight. The weight is thus on the feet and palms as the child balances.

72. SKIP

Skip for 40 or 50 feet, using right and left foot alternatively. This exercise helps to keep calcium in the bones.

73. SNOWMAN

Huge snowman, the sun comes out and he begins to melt. First his head, then his shoulders, then his waist begins to sag and his knees bend, then, very slowly he melts into the ground.

74. SORE TOE HOP

Each person hops down and back holding free foot in both hands.

75. SPARROW FIGHT

Two people in six-foot circle grasp own ankles

and try to oust opponent from circle.

76. STORK STAND

Stand on one foot, hands on hips. Balance body while placing one foot against inside of opposite leg. Change feet. Try with eyes closed for five seconds.

77. STORK WRESTLE

Standing on one leg, pull opponent off balance.

78. TABLES AND DISHES

Kneel on hands and knees with back level, making a flat table. On signal, hump the back, trying to throw all the dishes off. This is a good exercise for teaching abdominal control.

79. THREAD THE NEEDLE

Step through the circle formed by clasping hands, one leg at a time.

80. THREE AND ONE

Three players join hands and form a triangle, a fourth player stands outside facing the player opposite, and by dodging tries to touch him. The triangle must not be broken. All players should have a turn as catcher.

81. THROUGH TUG

Partners stand back to back and grasp right hand through their legs. They try to pull each other over a mark.

82. TIGHT ROPE WALK

Walk a line drawn on the floor (10 feet long). Use arms to balance.

83. TIN CAN STILTS

Each person goes down and back on stilts made from tin cans with strings tied to the sides.

84. TOE STEPPING

While keeping your own feet in constant motion, see who can be first to step on toes of opponent five times.

85. WALK TUNNEL

No. 1 stands in straddle position (feet apart), No. 2 crawls through and comes to a standing straddle position, and then No. 1 crawls through No. 2. Continue across room.

86. WAND PULL

Partners sit opposite each other with toes touching. Hold a wand or stick in centre, and partners try to pull each other off balance.

87. WASHING MACHINE

Feet apart, arms to sides – twisting vigorously from side to side.

88. WHEELBARROW

Number 1 grasps legs of Number 2 at knees

and walks as guiding a wheelbarrow. Number 2 walks on hands and keeps back straight.

89. **TRAFFIC**

Run, steer your own course – cars, aeroplanes, etc. Avoid each other.

90. **PARKING**

Run freely; stop, at signal, in a space. Run and find another space.

91. **TROTTING**

Run lightly and heavily, like ponies and carthorses.

92. **CHANGE DIRECTION**

Run listening for directions, turn, and stop, fast, slow, lightly, and heavily.

93. **SWAP**

Boys and girls on opposite sides of playground, change sides with various activities, galloping, giants, cars, engines, aeroplanes.

94. INVISI-BALL

Free run, on signal, jump high into the air as if to catch a ball, pull it in to the body.

95. REACH

Reach as high as possible in all directions.

96. CROSS

With feet wide apart, draw a big cross in the air with the hands.

97. CIRCLES

With feet wide apart, draw large circles with the head.

98. GIANTS

Like giants make large strides with the feet.

99. BIRD WALK

Take small, light, bouncing steps forward, with arms bent to imitate wings, like a bird walking.

100. FREESTYLE

Move around the ground any way you like, singly or with a partner - run, walk, hop, leap, slide or gallop.

Skipping Ropes

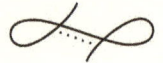

Skipping ropes can be made from polyurethane rope of suitable thickness available in hardware stores. Ropes should be of appropriate length and can be divided separately with a lighted candle. Don't let children do this work. Ropes with timber handles should not be used.

Jump rope (or skipping as it used to be called) is one of the best types of cardiovascular exercise there is. It is perfect for home use or to do while travelling, as ropes are inexpensive and easy to store.

Jump rope burns about one hundred calories in just

ten minutes, depending on your body weight. It also improves coordination and agility and tones both the upper and lower body.

Performance Guidelines for Teaching Methods

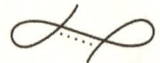

1. Teachers should always remember that their primary function is one of instruction and that instruction demands planning and organization.
2. Physical education instruction must proceed from the known to the unknown in a logical sequence.
3. Teachers should plan and conduct all instructional functions in the best interests of the students.
4. Concepts must be stressed so that students will know the 'why' of physical activity as well as the 'how'.

5. Teachers should inform students what they are about to learn and then evaluate in terms of the initial goals to determine teaching effectiveness.
6. Drills should as closely approximate the components of the actual game as possible. Drill for the sake of drill is irrelevant. Neuromuscular pathways are very specific; drills of a general nature should not be constructed.
7. Activities must be made interesting to be attractive to students.
8. Physical education should actively involve all the students in the class. The essence of the discipline is activity, not standing in lines. Adequate equipment and facility utilisation is imperative.
9. Teachers should always remain in a position whereby they can adequately supervise their students.
10. The class period in physical education should be primarily a period of instruction.

11. Teachers should strive to improve each student's skill according to the individual's capability, and set standards accordingly.

12. To be of real assistance, teachers must analyse the performance of each student and suggest measures necessary for improvement.

13. Praise and encouragement should be stressed; punishment should be used judiciously.

14. The use of instructional aides, either commercial or homemade, is encouraged as an adjunct to the teaching process.

15. Teachers should continually evaluate the instruction so that they become more efficient and effective in communicating information to students.

16. Performance Guidelines for Teaching Methods, Oregon State Department of Education, Salem, Oregon, 1979

Active Children better in the classroom

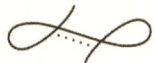

Children who get more exercise also tend to do better in school, whether the exercise comes as recess, physical education classes or getting exercise on the way to school, according to an international study. When researchers at the VU University Medical Center in Amsterdam asked students that those with higher rates of physical activity did better in the classroom. The study is published in the *Archives of Pediatrics & Adolescent Medicine*.

CPSIA information can be obtained
at www.ICGtesting.com
Printed in the USA
LVHW011952110122
708307LV00002B/86